300 Questions and Answers in Radiography and Fluid Therapy for Veterinary Nurses

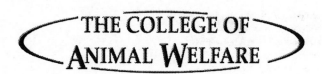

THE COLLEGE OF ANIMAL WELFARE

Senior commissioning editor: Mary Seager
Editorial assistant: Caroline Savage
Production controller: Anthony Read
Desk editor: Angela Davies
Cover designer: Helen Brockway

300 Questions and Answers in Radiography and Fluid Therapy for Veterinary Nurses

The College of Animal Welfare

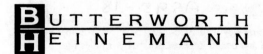

OXFORD   AUCKLAND   BOSTON
JOHANNESBURG   MELBOURNE   NEW DELHI

Butterworth-Heinemann
An imprint of Elsevier Science Limited

First published 2000
Reprinted 2002

British Library Cataloguing in Publication Data
300 questions and answers in radiology and fluid therapy. –
   (Veterinary nursing)
   1. Veterinary radiography – Examinations, questions, etc.
   2. Veterinary fluid therapy – Examinations, questions, etc.
   I.   College of Animal Welfare   II. Three hundred questions and
   answers in radiology and fluid therapy   III. Radiology and
   fluid therapy for veterinary nurses
   636'.089'607572'076

ISBN 0 7506 4794 9

Typeset by Keyword Typesetting Services, Wallington
Printed and bound in Great Britain by Biddles Ltd
www.biddles.co.uk

Contents

Acknowledgements   vi

Introduction   vii

Questions   1

Answers   82

Acknowledgements

The College is most grateful for the help of the following colleagues in the preparation of this book:

B. Cooper
B. Drysdale
D. Gould
J. Hargreaves
A. Jeffery
H. Orpet
A. Thomas
M. O'Reilly

Introduction

How the book is organized

This book of radiography and fluid therapy questions has been produced in response to further requests for more multiple choice questions. It contains 300 questions covering radiography and fluid therapy. After the questions is a list of correct answers.

How to use the book

Do your revision first, then select a range of question numbers at random. Do this without looking at the questions in advance. You should be able to complete and finish one multiple choice question per minute, allowing time for a thorough read of the question and the options before selecting the correct answer.

Questions

1) *What colour should a dark room be painted?*

   a) Black
   b) White
   c) Grey
   d) Beige

2) *The ideal temperature that a darkroom should be is:*

   a) 20–22°C
   b) 23–25°C
   c) 18–20°C
   d) 16–18°C

3) *The minimum distance that a direct safelight should be away from a work surface is:*

   a) 3 m
   b) 2 m
   c) 1.2 m
   d) 2.1 m

4) *Which bulb wattage would you use in a safelight?*
   a) 15 W
   b) 20 W
   c) 25 W
   d) 30 W

5) *The active ingredient in developer is:*
   a) ammonium thiosulphate
   b) calcium carbonate
   c) phenolic oxalate
   d) phenidone-hydroquinone

6) *The optimum temperature for a manual processing developer is:*
   a) 22°C
   b) 21°C
   c) 20°C
   d) 19°C

7) *The active ingredient in fixer is:*
   a) ammonium thiosulphate
   b) calcium carbonate
   c) phenolic oxalate
   d) phenidone-hydroquinone

8) *How long should a radiograph be washed for prior to drying?*

   a) 5–10 minutes
   b) 10–15 minutes
   c) 15–20 minutes
   d) 15–30 minutes

9) *What stage is omitted from an automatic processor?*

   a) Developer
   b) Rinse/stop bath
   c) Fixer
   d) Final wash

10) *At what temperature should automatic processing chemicals be kept?*

   a) 24°C
   b) 26°C
   c) 28°C
   d) 30°C

11) *What are the grains called that are on the film base and react with the light?*

   a) Gold halides
   b) Gold bromide
   c) Calcium halides
   d) Silver halides

12) *Non-screen film may be used for:*

   a) intra-oral views
   b) intracranial views
   c) intracardiac views
   d) intrahepatic views

13) *The phosphor calcium tungstate emits:*

   a) green light
   b) blue light
   c) red light
   d) yellow light

14) *Which ONE of the following is the BEST material for cleaning intensifying screens?*

   a) Cotton wool
   b) Tissue paper
   c) Swabs
   d) Nailbrush

15) *A fast film/screen combination requires:*

   a) more exposure
   b) less exposure
   c) an average exposure
   d) any of the above, because it makes no difference anyway

16) *A grid is placed:*

a) between the table and the cassette
b) between the x-ray beam and the patient
c) between the patient and the cassette
d) between the patient and the radiographer

17) *Tissue over a certain thickness should be x-rayed using a grid. What is this thickness?*

a) 40 cm
b) 15 cm
c) 20 cm
d) 10 cm

18) *Which legislation tells us that a patient should NOT be held for radiography, unless in exceptional circumstances?*

a) The Health and Safety at Work Act
b) The Control of Substances Hazardous to Health
c) The Ionising Radiation Regulations 1981
d) The Ionising Radiation Regulations 1999

19) *Scattered radiation increases with:*

a) an increased mA
b) a decreased mA
c) an increased kV
d) a decreased kV

20) *Which ONE of the following is used as a filter to stop low energy x-rays leaving the tube window?*

    a) Copper
    b) Lead
    c) Aluminium
    d) Tungsten

21) *The RPS (Radiation Protection Supervisor) is appointed:*

    a) within any practice involved with radiography
    b) outside the practice
    c) only if the practice takes more than 10 radiographs a week
    d) only if the practice has more than four people working there

22) *The RPA (Radiation Protection Advisor) is appointed:*

    a) within the practice
    b) outside the practice
    c) only if the practice takes more than 10 radiographs a week
    d) only if there are more than four people working in the practice

//////////||||||||||\\\\\\\\\\\\\\\\\

23) *The above grid is an example of a:*

   a) focused
   b) parallel
   c) pseudo-focused
   d) Potter Bucky

24) *Which ONE of the following people should NEVER be present during radiography?*

   a) 16–17 year olds
   b) People over the age of 18
   c) Over 21s
   d) Under 16 years of age

25) *Dosemeters should be worn:*

   a) on the shirt collar, outside a protective apron
   b) on the trunk, beneath a protective apron
   c) on the trunk, outside a protective apron
   d) on the shirt collar, beneath a protective apron

26) *The term medial describes a location:*

   a) towards the medial plane
   b) towards the tail
   c) towards the head
   d) away from the medial plane

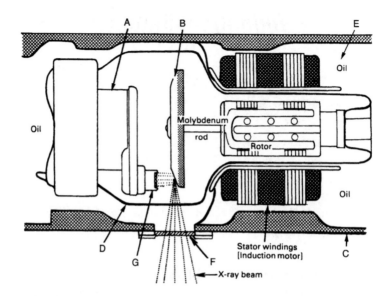

27) *The part labelled as 'E' is responsible for:*

   a) producing the electron beam
   b) preventing the moving electrons from colliding
      with air
   c) absorbing soft x-ray photons
   d) absorbing heat

28) *The part labelled 'F' on the tube head is the:*

   a) cathode
   b) aluminium filter
   c) filament
   d) x-ray beam

29) *The part labelled as 'G' is responsible for:*

 a) producing the electron beam
 b) preventing the moving electrons colliding with air
 c) absorbing soft x-ray photons
 d) absorbing heat

30) *The part labelled as 'B' is made of:*

 a) copper
 b) glass
 c) rhenium tungsten
 d) molybdenum

31) *When positioning for a BVA hip screen x-ray, where would you centre the primary beam?*

 a) On the wings of the ilium
 b) On the pubic symphysis
 c) On the acetabulum
 d) On the head of the femur

32) *Rostral describes a location:*

 a) away from the medial plane
 b) towards the tail
 c) towards the nose
 d) towards the head

33) *The phosphor calcium tungstate emits which colour light?*

   a) Green
   b) Blue
   c) Red
   d) Magenta

34) *Does a 'fast' film require a:*

   a) long exposure
   b) quick exposure
   c) medium exposure
   d) any of the above

35) *What is a latent image?*

   a) An image on the film after processing
   b) Calcium tungstate crystals in the film's emulsion that have been exposed to radiant energy before processing
   c) Silver halide crystals in the film's emulsion that have been exposed to radiant energy before processing
   d) An image on the film before processing

36) *A focused grid has:*

   a) both parallel and angled lead slats
   b) lead slats parallel to each other
   c) lead slats parallel to each other but getting smaller in size towards the edge of the grid
   d) lead slats that are at right angles to each to other

37) *A radiograph requires an exposure of 20 mA when taken at a film/focal distance of 90 cm without a grid. What exposure will be required if a grid with a grid factor of 4 is used?*

    a) 5 mA
    b) 30 mA
    c) 40 mA
    d) 80 mA

38) *Which ONE of the following is NOT an example of a phosphor used in intensifying screens?*

    a) Calcium tungstate
    b) Rare earth phosphors
    c) Barium lead sulphate
    d) Silver bromide

39) *The Radiation Protection Supervisor is usually:*

    a) a member of the practice, who is responsible for radiation safety but need not be present every time the x-ray machine is used
    b) a member of the practice, who is normally in charge of radiation safety and therefore must be present at every radiographic examination
    c) a veterinary surgeon who holds a diploma in veterinary radiography, and acts as an advisor in matters of radiation safety
    d) an external advisor, who can advise on radiation protection

40) *The target of an x-ray tube is usually made of:*

a) copper
b) lead
c) silver
d) tungsten

41) *What may cause a film to be too pale?*

a) Exhausted developer
b) Overexposure
c) Scattered radiation
d) Static electricity

42) *Which ONE of the following controls the quality or penetrating power of the x-ray beam?*

a) kV
b) mA
c) Time of exposure
d) All of the above

43) *Lead lined protective clothing is fully effective against:*

a) the primary beam and scattered radiation
b) the primary beam only
c) scattered radiation only
d) any sort of radiation at all

44) *Which ONE of the following items of equipment will reduce the risk of exposure to the primary beam?*

    a) Aluminium filter over the tube window
    b) Light beam diaphragm
    c) Protective clothing
    d) Rare earth screens

45) *Which ONE of the following will reduce the amount of scattered radiation reaching the film?*

    a) Increasing the film/focal distance
    b) Increasing the kV and decreasing the mA
    c) Reducing the exposure time and increasing the mA
    d) Reducing the size of the primary beam

46) *The old mA is 16. What will the new mA be given that the FFD is to be changed from 30 to 20?*

    a) 5 mA
    b) 6 mA
    c) 7 mA
    d) 8 mA

47) *An exposure for the radius of a GSD puppy was 30 kV, 10 mA. Unfortunately the puppy has a wet plaster of Paris cast on. What will the new exposure be?*

    a) 30 kV 20 mA
    b) 30 kV 40 mA
    c) 40 kV 10 mA
    d) 60 kV 10 mA

48) *An exposure for a Labrador is 50 kV and 15 mA.*
     However, a grid with a factor of 2 is to be used. What
     will the new exposure be?

     a) 50 kV $7\frac{1}{2}$ mA
     b) 100 kV 15 mA
     c) 50 kV 30 mA
     d) 100 kV 30 mA

49) *If the kV is raised by 10 to 70 kV and the mA is 20*
     what effect will this have on the exposure?

     a) 70 kV and 10 mA
     b) 70 kV and 40 mA
     c) 80 kV and 20 mA
     d) 80 kV and 60 mA

50) *What will the exposure be if the FFD is changed from*
     75 cm to 90 cm with an old mA of 20?

     a) 16
     b) 16.67
     c) 24.0
     d) 28.8

51) *An exposure of 60 kV and 40 mA using a grid with a*
     factor of 2 has proved successful. What will the
     exposure be if the grid is removed?

     a) 10 mA
     b) 20 mA
     c) 60 mA
     d) 80 mA

52) *What will the exposure time be for an exposure of 15 mAs with the mA at 10?*

    a) 1 second
    b) 1.5 seconds
    c) 2 seconds
    d) 3 seconds

53) *Which ONE of the following is an example of a water soluble positive contrast agent?*

    a) Barium sulphate
    b) Air
    c) Carbon dioxide
    d) Iodine

54) *Who is responsible for writing the Radiographic Local Rules?*

    a) The senior partner
    b) The RPA
    c) The RPS
    d) The head nurse

55) *In a typical practice the controlled area is within a _____ radius from the primary beam*

    a) 6 metres
    b) 4 metres
    c) 2 metres
    d) 0.5 metres

56) *Which ONE of the following imaging techniques CANNOT be used for skeletal investigations?*

   a) Ultrasonography
   b) CT scanning
   c) Magnetic resonance imaging
   d) Scintigraphy

57) *Inherited abnormalities caused by radiography are due to:*

   a) somatic effects
   b) genetic effect
   c) carcinogenic effects
   d) cumulative effect

58) *A film that is too dark may be as a result of:*

   a) FFD too short
   b) underexposure
   c) underdevelopment
   d) FFD too long

59) *The term soot and whitewash may be used to describe a film where:*

   a) the developer was not stirred
   b) overexposure has occurred
   c) the kilovoltage is too low
   d) fogging has occurred

60) *Dirty intensifying screens will result in:*

   a) yellow stains on the film
   b) borders around the film
   c) fogging
   d) small bright marks on the film

61) *Which ONE of the following is responsible for image blurring?*

   a) Patient movement
   b) Scattered radiation
   c) FFD too long
   d) Fogging

62) *What remedial action would you NOT take to prevent fogging?*

   a) Collimate beam
   b) Increase kilovoltage
   c) Use a grid
   d) Use films before expiry date

63) *Black crescent marks may be prevented by:*

   a) correct washing procedure
   b) use anti-static screen cleaner
   c) careful handling of unprocessed film
   d) cleaning the rollers of the automatic processor

64) *The minimum standard of lead equivalent for protective gloves and sleeves is:*

a) 0.30 mm equivalent
b) 0.35 mm equivalent
c) 0.20 mm equivalent
d) 0.25 mm equivalent

65) *Radiographic density is determined by the:*

a) exposure factor
b) exposure factor and processing technique
c) processing technique
d) focal film distance

66) *Which ONE of the following statements concerning positioning for radiography is NOT true?*

a) Exposures of the abdomen should always be taken on inspiration
b) Exposures of the chest should always be taken on inspiration
c) The nasal chambers are best viewed using an intra-oral film
d) To examine the heart, a D/V view is more useful than a V/D view, as in the latter the heart may tip to one side

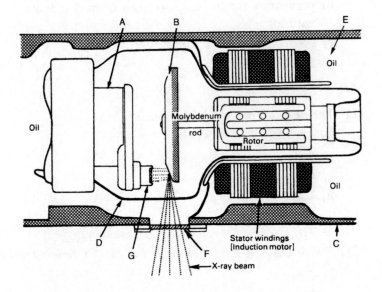

67) *The above grid is an example of a:*

   a) Parallel grid
   b) Focused grid
   c) Pseudo- focused grid
   d) Potter Bucky

68) *The part labelled as 'A' on the stationary x-ray tube is the:*

   a) anode
   b) cathode
   c) cooling fins
   d) focusing cup

69) *The part labelled as 'B' is the:*

   a) the anode
   b) the cathode
   c) the cooling fins
   d) the aluminium filter

70) *The part labelled as 'C' is responsible for:*

   a) producing the electron beam
   b) preventing the moving electrons from colliding with air
   c) absorbing soft x-ray photons
   d) absorbing heat

71) *The part labelled as 'D' is made of:*

   a) copper
   b) glass
   c) rhenium tungsten
   d) molybdenum

72) *Which ONE of the following is the MOST radiopaque?*

   a) Gas
   b) Bone
   c) Fat
   d) Soft tissue

73) *The degree of absorption by a given tissue does NOT depend on:*

   a) the atomic number
   b) the specific gravity of the tissue
   c) thickness of the tissue
   d) the milliamperage

74) *Positively charged particles contained in the centre of an atom are known as:*

   a) electrons
   b) photons
   c) neutrons
   d) protons

75) *The height of the strips to the width of the radiolucent interspace in a grid is known as the:*

   a) grid factor
   b) grid ratio
   c) grid lines
   d) grid number

76) *Film that is both blue and green light sensitive is known as:*

   a) monochromatic
   b) non-screen
   c) orthochromatic
   d) ultraviolet

77) *The developer contains a restrainer to:*
   a) reduce the amount of developmental fog
   b) maintain alkalinity of the solution
   c) maintain the acidity of the solution
   d) prevent oxidation

78) *If the FFD is too long the resultant image will be:*
   a) blurred
   b) too dark
   c) too pale
   d) fogged

79) *Which ONE is not a remedial action for a film that is too pale?*
   a) Increase temperature of developer
   b) Change developer
   c) Increase exposure
   d) Increase FFD

80) *Fogging is NOT caused by:*
   a) scatter from the table
   b) scatter from the patient
   c) developer not stirred
   d) exposure to white light before fixing

81) *Which ONE of the following is NOT a danger associated with radiography?*

   a) Visible
   b) Painless
   c) Latent
   d) Cumulative

82) *Which technique would be used to demonstrate a joint space?*

   a) Fistulography
   b) Arthrography
   c) Bronchography
   d) Venography

83) *The quantity of x-rays produced depends upon:*

   a) milliamperage
   b) length of the exposure
   c) both a and b
   d) kilovoltage

84) *Which ONE of the following will NOT reduce scatter radiation?*

   a) Collimation of the beam
   b) Compression band
   c) Increase kV
   d) Grid

85) *Blurring of one part of the film will occur due to:*

   a) poor screen–film contact
   b) underexposure
   c) overexposure
   d) FFD too long

86) *Which ONE of the following is the most radiolucent?*

   a) Metal
   b) Bone
   c) Fat
   d) Soft tissue

87) *Which combination will give you the best definition?*

   a) Fast film, fast screen
   b) Fast film, slow screen
   c) Slow film, fast screen
   d) Slow film, slow screen

88) *Which ONE of the following techniques is most likely to be used for fine needle aspiration of the liver?*

   a) Computed tomography
   b) Magnetic resonance imaging
   c) Scintigraphy
   d) Ultrasound

89) *Which ONE of the following is NOT a requirement for films submitted to BVA/Kennel Club Hip Dysplasia Scoring Scheme?*

    a) Patient's Kennel Club number
    b) Dog's name
    c) Date
    d) Left marker

90) *Which ONE of the following affects the quality of the x-ray beam?*

    a) The kilovoltage
    b) The milliamperage
    c) Time
    d) The tube rating

91) *What would the mA be if the FFD was altered from 75 cm to 100 cm assuming that the currect mA is 30?*

    a) 30 mA
    b) 60 mA
    c) 50 mA
    d) 70 mA

92) *To maintain the same exposure, what would the mA be if the kV was increased by 10? Current exposure used is 20 kV 30 mA.*

    a) 20 kV 10 mA
    b) 30 kV 15 mA
    c) 30 kV 20 mA
    d) 30 kV 20 mA

93) *White patches on a film may be caused by:*
   a) water splashes onto film before processing
   b) developer splashes onto film before processing
   c) insufficient washing
   d) fixer splashes onto film before processing

94) *Which ONE of the following has a higher atomic number than bone?*
   a) Gas
   b) Fat
   c) Soft tissue
   d) Metal

95) *Blackening of the film is caused by the:*
   a) kilovoltage
   b) milliamperage
   c) increased FFD
   d) kilovoltage and milliamperage

96) *Electrons are:*
   a) negatively charged particles which orbit the nucleus
   b) positively charged particles in the nucleus
   c) particles of similar size to protons but carry no charge
   d) combination of two or more elements

97) *The maximum dose of radiation a member of the general public (over 18) may legally receive to the whole body in a year is:*

   a) no dose at all
   b) 5 mSv
   c) 15 mSv
   d) 50 mSv

98) *The use of x-rays in practice is controlled by which piece of legislation?*

   a) Health & Safety at Work Act
   b) COSHH Regulation
   c) Guidance Notes for the Protection of Persons against Ionising Radiations arising from Veterinary use
   d) Ionising Radiation Regulations

99) *By using which ONE of the following techniques could you reduce radiation hazards by the greatest amount?*

   a) Increasing the kV
   b) Reducing film/focus distance
   c) Use of the grid
   d) Use of the rare earth screens

100) *Which ONE of the following affects radiographic contrast?*

a) kV
b) mA
c) Use of a grid
d) All of the above

101) *Which ONE of the following procedures will help to improve the definition of an x-ray image by the greatest amount?*

a) Use of a non-screen film
b) Decreasing film/focal distance
c) Increasing film/focal distance
d) Increasing the kV

102) *An x-ray film that you have processed is too dark. How would you correct this error?*

a) Increase development time
b) Increase the kV
c) Reduce the exposure time
d) Reduce the film/focal time

103) *A processed film is very grey with poor contrast between the image and the background. What could be the cause?*

a) kV too high
b) Film fogged by radiation
c) Exhausted developer
d) Developer temperature too high

104) *A radiograph of an anaesthetised animal is blurred.*
     What might be the cause?

   a) Exhausted developer
   b) Inadequate fixing
   c) Poor film/screen contact
   d) Underexposure

105) *What mark or artefact would insufficient washing after*
     fixation leave on a finished radiograph?

   a) White spots
   b) Dark spots
   c) Yellow stains
   d) Cloudy appearance

106) *Which are the two major components of an x-ray film*
     emulsion?

   a) Gelatin and silver halides
   b) Gelatin and silver ions
   c) Silver ions and silver halides
   d) Gelatin and silver oxide

107) *The filament of an x-ray tube is normally made of:*

   a) copper
   b) lead
   c) silver
   d) tungsten

108) *When taking a radiograph for the BVA/Kennel Club Hip Dysplasia Scoring Scheme, what information must be included on the radiograph?*

   a) Dog's name, KC number, L/R marker
   b) KC number, date, L/R marker
   c) KC number, L/R marker
   d) Practice name and address, dog's name, L/R marker

109) *In which ONE of the following positions should a dog be placed following a myelogram?*

   a) Head elevated about 30 degrees
   b) Normal recovery position
   c) The head lowered below the rest of the body
   d) Sternal recumbency

110) *Which ONE of the following is NOT an advantage of rare earth screens?*

   a) Increased exposure time
   b) Decreased patient dose
   c) Improved image quality
   d) Reduced tube current

111) *Which film fault is responsible for white spots on the radiograph?*

   a) Dirt on the intensifying screens
   b) Film not agitated sufficiently
   c) Fixer splashed onto the film before processing
   d) Film underdeveloped

112) *Which ONE of the following chemicals is NOT a constituent of the fixer?*

   a) Ammonium thiosulphate
   b) Boric acid
   c) Potassium bromide
   d) Sodium acetate

113) *Which is the 'fixing agent' used in a fixer?*

   a) Ammonium chloride
   b) Ammonium thiosulphate
   c) Potassium hydroxide
   d) Sodium acetate

114) *Which ONE of the following is removed from the film during fixing?*

   a) Ammonium thiosulphate
   b) Silver halide
   c) Silver nitrate
   d) Sodium chloride

115) *Where would you find an intensifying screen?*

   a) In a grid
   b) In an x-ray cassette
   c) On the wall (used to illuminate x-rays for viewing)
   d) In the developing tank

116) *You have developed a radiograph using the wet tank method, and the film has turned out yellow. What is this due to?*

a) Contamination of the developer
b) Exhausted developer
c) Fixer being spilt on the film before processing
d) Fixing time too short

117) *When taking a ventro-dorsal radiograph of the cervical spine, the disc spaces will be viewed most accurately if:*

a) the forelimbs are pulled forwards, towards the animal's head
b) the neck is supported with sandbags
c) the tube head is inclined 15–20 degrees towards the head
d) the tube head is inclined 15–20 degrees towards the thorax

118) *When positioning a dog for a BVA/Kennel Club hip radiograph, the beam should be centred on:*

a) the acetabula
b) the pubic symphysis
c) the sacrum
d) the wings of the ilium

119) *Use of rare earth screens may decrease exposure factors or time by up to:*

    a) 10%
    b) 30%
    c) 70%
    d) 90%

120) *The speed of the intensifying screen is increased by:*

    a) a thick fluorescent layer of large crystals
    b) a thick fluorescent layer of small crystals
    c) a thin fluorescent layer of large crystals
    d) a thin fluorescent layer of small crystals

121) *What effect will faster speed have on the definition of the film image?*

    a) Increased
    b) Decreased
    c) Magnified
    d) Unaffected

122) *What is the exposure fault of a radiograph with a pale image, of HIGH contrast, on a dark background?*

    a) kV too low
    b) kV too high
    c) mA too low
    d) mA too high

123) *The use of a grid requires an increase in the:*

    a) milliamperage/second
    b) kilovoltage
    c) film focal distance
    d) collimation

124) *The latent image of the exposed radiation is the result of:*

    a) the developing process
    b) the fixing process
    c) exposure to light/x-ray photons
    d) scatter radiation

125) *If you were developing non-screen film manually, how much longer would you leave the film in the developer compared to screen film?*

    a) Double the normal developing time
    b) Increase by 2 minutes
    c) Same time as normal film
    d) Increase by 30 seconds

126) *Which ONE of the following crystals may be found in the 'rare earth' screens?*

    a) Calcium tungstate
    b) Silver bromide
    c) Silver thiosulphate
    d) Gadolinium oxysulphide

127) *Which ONE of the following exposure functions affects the amount of x-rays produced?*

   a) kV
   b) mA
   c) FFD
   d) Time

128) *The reflective layer of the intensifying screens is:*

   a) required to filter out scatter radiation
   b) between the film and the fluorescent layer
   c) to prevent back scatter reaching the film
   d) to reflect light photons back towards the film

129) *The visible difference between varying shades (tones) of the film image is called the:*

   a) density
   b) contrast
   c) definition
   d) clarity

130) *X-rays are members of the:*

   a) electro-magnetic spectrum
   b) radio wave spectrum
   c) electro-radiation spectrum
   d) radio frequency spectrum

131) *The cloud of electrons is produced at the:*

   a) anode
   b) cathode
   c) anion
   d) cation

132) *How much electron energy is lost via heat production?*

   a) 20%
   b) 1%
   c) 99%
   d) 25%

133) *What is the filter made of that the x-rays have to pass through when leaving the tube head?*

   a) Copper
   b) Tungsten
   c) Lead
   d) Aluminium

134) *The anode is:*

   a) positively charged
   b) negatively charged
   c) inversely charged
   d) all of the above

135) *The target (anode) is set at which angle?*

   a) 20°
   b) 25°
   c) 30°
   d) 35°

136) *What does kV control?*

   a) Penetration power
   b) Quality
   c) Speed
   d) Exposure time

137) *Which ONE of the following would NOT reduce fogging?*

   a) Collimate beam
   b) Use of a grid
   c) Correct development technique
   d) Prolonged storage

138) *Which ONE of the following grid types will NOT result in the presence of visible parallel lines on a radiograph?*

   a) Potter Bucky
   b) Focused
   c) Parallel
   d) Psuedo-focused

139) *Which crystals do thermo-luminescent dosemeters contain?*

   a) Oxalate fluoride
   b) Lithium fluoride
   c) Ammonium fluoride
   d) Calcium fluoride

140) *Which ONE of the following is not a usual layer of x-ray film?*

   a) Subbing layer
   b) Protective supercoat
   c) Polyester base
   d) Anti-halation backing

141) *Increasing the mA on an x-ray machine increases:*

   a) the penetration power of the x-ray beam
   b) the amount of electrons produced by the cathode
   c) the speed at which the electrons are accelerated across the vacuum
   d) the length of time that the film is exposed to the x-ray film

142) *The exposure for a lateral chest x-ray has 60 kV 16 mA at a film focal distance (FFD) of 75 cm. Which one of the following exposures is the correct mA if the FFD is changed to 60 cm?*

    a) 8 mA
    b) 10 mA
    c) 12 mA
    d) 14 mA

143) *Too high a kV produces:*

    a) a film low in contrast
    b) a film low in density
    c) a film high in contrast
    d) a film high in density

144) *The absorption of x-rays by a tissue depends on which ONE of the following?*

    a) Atomic number
    b) Density of tissue
    c) Thickness of tissue
    d) All of the above

145) *Which one of the following is NOT a property of x-rays?*

    a) They are not reflected
    b) They can cause fluorescence of certain materials
    c) They do not travel in straight lines
    d) They show different rates of absorption

146) *Gas on a radiograph will show up as:*

   a) white
   b) dark grey
   c) mid-grey
   d) nearly black

147) *Soft tissue on a radiograph will show up as:*

   a) white
   b) dark grey
   c) mid-grey
   d) nearly black

148) *Underdevelopment of a film will produce an x-ray that is:*

   a) too pale
   b) too dark
   c) of too high contrast
   d) of little definition

149) *Which ONE of the following is NOT a cause of film fogging?*

   a) Exposure to scatter
   b) Overdevelopment
   c) Too low a safelight wattage
   d) Chemical fumes

150) *The exposure for a radiograph of the left femur is 55 kV, 22 mA at a film focal distance (FFD) of 80 cm. Which ONE of the following is the correct mA if the FFD if changed to 95 cm?*

a) 25 mA
b) 27 mA
c) 29 mA
d) 31 mA

151) *Which ONE of the following types of anode produces limited x-ray production?*

a) Rotating anode
b) Stationary anode
c) Revolving anode
d) Oscillating anode

152) *The envelope that contains the anode and cathode is made from:*

a) perspex
b) pyrex
c) aluminium
d) lead

153) *The focusing cup in an x-ray tube head is COMMONLY made from which one of the following metals?*

   a) Nickel
   b) Copper
   c) Tungsten
   d) Lead

154) *The anode is made from which ONE of the following metals?*

   a) Nickel
   b) Copper
   c) Tungsten
   d) Lead

155) *The anode of the x-ray tube head attracts:*

   a) protons
   b) atoms
   c) neutrons
   d) electrons

156) *1% of the energy used in a tube head creates x-rays, the other 99% of the energy is converted into:*

   a) kinetic energy
   b) heat
   c) monochromatic light
   d) orthochromatic light

157) *In a stationary anode, the target is embedded in a stem of:*

   a) nickel
   b) tungsten
   c) copper
   d) lead

158) *The usable x-ray beam comes from an area of the anode called the:*

   a) effective focal spot
   b) inverse focal spot
   c) actual focal spot
   d) opposing focal spot

159) *Which ONE of the following does kV (kilovoltage) NOT control?*

   a) The speed at which the electrons travel
   b) The quantity of electrons produced at the cathode
   c) The penetration power of the x-ray beam
   d) The energy of the electrons

160) *Which ONE of the following is the light sensitive part of the x-ray film emulsion?*

   a) Silver halide crystals
   b) Potassium bromide crystals
   c) Potassium silver crystals
   d) Silver-potassium crystals

161) *Which ONE of the following film types is sensitive to green light?*

   a) Orthochromatic film
   b) Polychromatic film
   c) Monochromatic film
   d) Trichromatic film

162) *Which ONE of the following radiographic studies would you use non-screen film for?*

   a) Lateral view of a femur
   b) Caudo-cranial view of the stifle
   c) Dorso-ventral view of the internal nares
   d) Lateral thorax

163) *The phosphor calcium tungstate emits which colour of light when it fluoresces?*

   a) Green
   b) Blue
   c) Cyan
   d) Magenta

164) *Which ONE of the following is NOT an advantage of using intensifying screens?*

   a) Reduced exposure time
   b) Increased tube current
   c) Reduced movement blur
   d) Decreased tube voltage

165) *Fast screen–film combinations:*

a) have large silver halide crystals and large screen phosphor crystals
b) have small silver halide crystals and small screen phosphor crystals
c) have small silver nitrate crystals and small screen phosphor crystals
d) have small silver halide crystals and large screen phosphor crystals

166) *Slow screen–film combinations:*

a) have large silver halide crystals and large screen phosphor crystals
b) have small silver halide crystals and small screen phosphor crystals
c) have small silver nitrate crystals and small screen phosphor crystals
d) have small silver halide crystals and large screen phosphor crystals

167) *Which ONE of the following is NOT true about intensifying screens?*

a) They reduce exposure time
b) They reduce the overall definition of the finished radiograph
c) They are used singly
d) They are very fragile and easily damaged

168) *Screen–film contact can be checked by:*

a) placing paper clips inside an x-ray cassette, exposing the film briefly to the primary beam and then processing the film

b) placing chicken wire over the x-ray cassette, exposing the film briefly to the primary beam and then processing the film

c) placing chicken wire over the x-ray cassette, then allowing the cassette to be exposed to white light over a period of time and then processing it

d) placing paper clips on the outside of the cassette, exposing the cassette to the darkroom safelight for 10 minutes and then processing the film

169) *Which ONE of the following terms best describes the term 'distally'?*

a) Towards the head

b) Towards the tail

c) Away from the nose

d) Away from the site of attachment

170) *If a proprietary brand of screen/cassette cleaner is NOT available, which ONE of the following products would be the best?*

a) Hibiscrub

b) Water

c) Pevidine

d) Saline

171) *After cleaning an x-ray cassette, what is the best way to leave it to dry?*

   a) Open, standing upright (like a book)
   b) Open, laying flat
   c) Completely closed, laying flat
   d) Partially closed, but next to a window so it dries quickly

172) *Which ONE of the following is NOT a function of an x-ray cassette?*

   a) To hold the intensifying screens and protect them from damage
   b) To exclude all light from the cassette
   c) To maintain a close and uniform contact between the screens and the films
   d) To help insulate the animal whilst it is undergoing a radiographic examination

173) *Which ONE of the following is x-ray film not sensitive to?*

   a) Gamma rays
   b) Radio waves
   c) Ultra-violet light
   d) Pressure

174) *A fast film requires:*

    a) a long exposure time
    b) a short exposure time
    c) an average exposure time
    d) any of the above, it doesn't matter

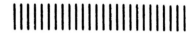

175) *The above grid is an example of what type of grid?*

    a) Focused
    b) Parallel
    c) Potter Bucky
    d) Pseudo-focused

176) *Grids are useful at absorbing:*

    a) scattered radiation
    b) the primary beam
    c) any stray white light that might be present during the exposure
    d) any stray gamma rays that might be around during the exposure

177) *Which ONE of the following is a moving grid?*

    a) A parallel grid
    b) A crossed grid
    c) A Potter Bucky diaphragm
    d) A pseudo-focused grid

178) *Which ONE of the following is the least expensive type of grid?*

    a) A parallel grid
    b) A crossed grid
    c) A focused grid
    d) A pseudo-focused grid

179) *The term used to describe the unprocessed image on an x-ray film is:*

    a) latent image
    b) occluded image
    c) superimposed image
    d) obscured image

180) *The usual time an x-ray film needs to be processed for is:*

    a) 1 minute
    b) 1–2 minutes
    c) 3–5 minutes
    d) 6–7 minutes

181) *Developer is:*

    a) strongly acidic
    b) mildly acidic
    c) neutral
    d) alkaline

182) *A common chemical used as the 'stopping' agent is:*

   a) acetic acid
   b) acetic trisulphate
   c) metol-hydroquinone
   d) bromide–chloride

183) *'Fixing' a film is done for which ONE of the following reasons?*

   a) To dissolve and remove the exposed silver halides from the x-ray film
   b) To dissolve and remove the unexposed silver halides from the x-ray film
   c) To dissolve and remove the anti-halation backing from the film
   d) To soften the emulsion: making it easier to wash and dry

184) *The emulsion of non-screen film is thicker than that of screen film. Which one of the following changes would you make to the processing time?*

   a) Increase the development time and decrease the fixing time
   b) Increase the development time and increase the fixing time
   c) Decrease the development time and increase the fixing time
   d) Decrease the development time and decrease the fixing time

185) *The accelerator 'potassium carbonate' is often included in developer to:*

a) decrease the amount of developmental fog
b) decrease the time it takes for developer to oxidise
c) increase the hardness of the film emulsion
d) increase the alkalinity of the developer

186) *Preservatives are included in the developer to:*

a) decrease the amount of developmental fog
b) slow down the time it takes for the developer to oxidise
c) increase the hardness of the film emulsion
d) increase the alkalinity of the developer

187) *Restrainers are included in the developer to:*

a) decrease the amount of developmental fog
b) decrease the time it takes for developer to oxidise
c) increase the hardness of the film emulsion
d) increase the alkalinity of the developer

188) *A COMMON preservative in fixer is:*

a) sodium thiosulphate
b) sodium sulphite
c) sodium carbonate
d) ammonium sulphite

189) *A radiograph can be viewed briefly in the dark room after approximately how long in the fixer?*

   a) 30 seconds
   b) 2 minutes
   c) 5 minutes
   d) 1 minute

190) *Buffers are included in the fixer to:*

   a) increase the pH of the fixer
   b) decrease the pH of the fixer
   c) maintain the pH of the fixer
   d) speed up the fixing process

191) *How long should a processed radiograph be washed for in circulating water?*

   a) 60 minutes
   b) 45 minutes
   c) 30–40 minutes
   d) 20–30 minutes

192) *Which ONE of the following is NOT a method of silver recovery?*

   a) Metallic replacement
   b) Electrolytic recovery
   c) Chemical precipitation
   d) Electro-magnetic recovery

193) *Lateral radiographs should be viewed so that:*

   a) the spine runs parallel to the top of the light box and the head points towards viewer's left hand side
   b) the spine runs vertically to the top of the light box and the head points towards the viewer's right hand side
   c) the spine runs parallel to the top of the light box, with the head pointing uppermost
   d) the spine runs vertically to the top of the light box, with the head pointing downwards

194) *The 'subbing layer' of a piece of x-ray film could also be called the:*

   a) adhesive layer
   b) emulsion layer
   c) protective layer
   d) film base

195) *What is the minimum lead equivalent (LE) of an apron?*

   a) 0.25 mm LE
   b) 0.35 mm LE
   c) 0.5 mm LE
   d) 0.6 mm LE

196) *Which ONE of the following substances is commonly used in protective clothing?*

   a) Tungsten
   b) Lead
   c) Aluminium
   d) Copper

197) *Which ONE of the following imaging techniques produces cross-sectional views of a patient's body?*

   a) Fluoroscopy
   b) Computed tomography
   c) Radionuclide imaging
   d) Ultrasound scanning

198) *Which ONE of the following imaging techniques involves the patient having a radioactive isotope introduced to the body?*

   a) Fluoroscopy
   b) Computed tomography
   c) Radionuclide imaging
   d) Ultrasound scanning

199) *Which ONE of the following studies would you use the contrast medium barium sulphate for?*

   a) Cardioangiography
   b) Intravenous urography
   c) Sialography
   d) Gastrography

200) *Which ONE of the following is a non-ionic water-soluble iodine contrast medium?*

   a) Sodium iothalmate
   b) Sodium ioxaglate
   c) Iopamidol
   d) Sodium diatrizoate

201) *X-rays and gamma rays are:*

   a) high in frequency, long in wavelength
   b) low in frequency, short in wavelength
   c) high in frequency, medium in wavelength
   d) high in frequency, short in wavelength

202) *X-rays are produced by:*

   a) decay of radioactive material
   b) x-ray machines
   c) radon gas
   d) a chemical compound

203) *X-rays are produced when fast moving _____ hit a target at high speed*

   a) Protons
   b) Neutrons
   c) Atoms
   d) Electrons

204) *Kinetic energy is:*
   a) energy produced by movement
   b) energy produced by sound
   c) energy produced by light
   d) energy produced by heat

205) *The 'high potential difference' is measured in:*
   a) milliamperes
   b) kilovolts
   c) kilowatts
   d) megahertz

206) *Which ONE of the following is positively charged?*
   a) Anode
   b) Focusing cup
   c) Wire filament
   d) Cathode

207) *What percentage of energy is lost in heat production?*
   a) 1%
   b) 9%
   c) 79%
   d) 99%

208) *What is the filter made of through which all x-rays have to pass, prior to leaving the tube head?*

   a) Tungsten
   b) Copper
   c) Aluminium
   d) Lead

209) *Which ONE of the following metals lines the tube head?*

   a) Tungsten
   b) Copper
   c) Aluminium
   d) Lead

210) *Which ONE of the following gases is not used in contrast studies*

   a) Carbon dioxide
   b) Room air
   c) Oxygen
   d) Carbon monoxide

211) *Which ONE of the following contrast media should be used for myelograms?*

   a) Sodium iothalmate
   b) Iopamidol
   c) Sodium ioxaglate
   d) Sodium diatrizoate

212) *Which ONE of the following offers the least protection against ionising radiation?*

   a) Double sided, x-ray gown
   b) Leaded glasses
   c) Dosemeter
   d) Cassette holder

213) *Which ONE of the following methods of patient restraint offers the greatest protection from radiation exposure?*

   a) Sedation, without holding the patient
   b) Rope ties, held at a distance
   c) Lead sleeves, held away from the primary beam
   d) Full-leaded gloves, apron

214) *Which ONE of the following parts of the x-ray machine limits primary beam size and lessens secondary radiation exposure to personnel?*

   a) Aluminium filter
   b) Line voltage compensator
   c) Light beam diaphragm
   d) Lead-lined tube head

215) *Which ONE of the following gives an increased chance of being exposed to ionising radiation?*

   a) Increased tube voltage
   b) Repeated exposures
   c) Longer film focal distance
   d) Using a Potter Bucky diaphragm

216) *If a radiographer doubles his/her distance from the primary beam, e.g. moves from 2 metres to 4 metres, which one of the following would be the dose of radiation that they received?*

   a) 1/5
   b) 1/4
   c) 1/2
   d) 1/10

217) *Which one of the following times is it acceptable to have part of your body in contact with the primary beam?*

   a) When your hands are protected with lead gloves
   b) When a patient is too ill to be restrained in any other way, e.g. a ruptured diaphragm
   c) When a large animal x-ray needs to be taken and there is no other way of supporting the x-ray other than by holding it.
   d) None of the above, it is never acceptable to have part of your body exposed to the primary beam.

218) *What is the cause of dark 'branches' running across a processed radiograph?*

   a) Static electricity that has been discharged during film handling
   b) Developer time is too quick
   c) Somebody opening the cassette and exposing the film to white light briefly
   d) Too great an exposure of the film to the safelight

219) *Which ONE of the following would decrease the likelihood of radiographs turning yellow over a period of time?*

   a) Allowing more time for the radiograph to be fixed
   b) Allowing more time for the radiograph to be washed
   c) Decreasing the time the radiograph spends in the developer
   d) Increasing the time that the radiograph is in the stop bath

220) *Which ONE of the following safelight filters is commonly used when handling orthochromatic film?*

   a) Dark brown
   b) Yellow brown
   c) Dark green
   d) Dark red

221) *Which ONE of the following safelight filters is used when handling monochromatic film?*

   a) Dark red
   b) Dark green
   c) Brown
   d) Blue

222) *Which ONE of the following is the main source of scattered radiation?*

    a) Cathode
    b) Patient
    c) Anode
    d) Cassette

223) *Which is the correct sequence when processing a film manually?*

    a) Develop, fix, wash, dry
    b) Fix, wash, develop, stop, dry
    c) Develop, stop, fix, wash, dry
    d) Wash, develop, stop, fix, dry

224) *Which ONE of the following is the correct sequence when using an automatic processor?*

    a) Develop, fix, wash, dry
    b) Fix, wash, developer, stop, dry
    c) Develop, stop, fix, wash, dry
    d) Wash, develop, stop, fix, dry

225) *If you increase the film to object distance, then the image is:*

    a) magnified
    b) blurred
    c) lighter
    d) darker

226) *Which ONE of the following terms BEST describes the distance from the tube head to the film cassette?*

a) Focal object
b) Object–film distance
c) Effective focal distance
d) Film focal distance

227) *If the mA is 60 and the seconds is 0.2, what should the mAs be set to?*

a) 12
b) 9
c) 6
d) 3

228) *When calculating exposure times, if the mA is 50 and the time is 0.25 seconds, what should the mAs be set to?*

a) 8.5
b) 10
c) 12.5
d) 14

229) *Dichroic fog is caused by:*

a) exhausted developer
b) static electricity
c) insufficient washing
d) scattered radiation

230) *Patchy film density may be caused by:*

   a) film is not agitated in developer
   b) exhausted filter
   c) kV too low
   d) fogging

231) *Yellow-brown patches may occur as a result of:*

   a) exhausted developer
   b) insufficient fixing
   c) overdevelopment
   d) chemical splashes on film

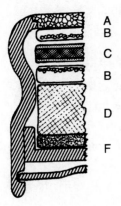

232) *What is part 'A' on the exploded section of the x-ray cassette?*

   a) Radiolucent front
   b) X-ray film
   c) Back screen
   d) Lead backing

233) *The purpose of 'E' is to:*

a) intensify the effect of x-rays
b) produce the image
c) absorb remaining x-rays and absorb scatter
d) ensure close contact between the film and the screens

234) *What is part 'F' on the exploded section of the x-ray cassette?*

a) Front screen
b) X-ray film
c) Back screen
d) Lead backing

235) *The purpose of 'B' is to:*

a) intensify the effect of x-rays
b) produce the image
c) absorb x-rays
d) ensure close contact between the film and the screens

236) *Which layer is responsible for forming the image on the picture of the x-ray cassette?*

a) A
b) C
c) D
d) F

237) *'C' on the picture of an x-ray cassette consists of a material containing:*

a) calcium tungstate
b) phosphor
c) silver bromide
d) lead

238) *Which ONE of the following is NOT responsible for image blurring?*

a) Patient movement
b) Scattered radiation
c) Fogging
d) Insufficient washing

239) *Which ONE of the following is NOT responsible for fogging an x-ray image?*

a) Underexposure
b) Exposure to white light before fixing
c) Scattered radiation from the patient
d) Prolonged storage

240) *Insufficient washing of an x-ray film may give rise to:*

a) fogging
b) pink-green stains
c) blurring
d) soot and whitewash appearance

241) *When measuring urine output during canine surgery which ONE of the following would be an acceptable minimum output?*

   a) 7–8 ml/kg/h
   b) 5–6 ml/kg/h
   c) 3–4 ml/kg/h
   d) 1–2 ml/kg/h

242) *A 20-kg dog needs 60 ml/h infusion with a standard drip set. Which of the following would be correct?*

   a) 1 drop/3 seconds
   b) 3 drops/1 second
   c) 6 drops/1 second
   d) 1 drop/6 seconds

243) *How much of a newborn animal's body weight is water?*

   a) 25–30%
   b) 30–40%
   c) 50–60%
   d) 75–80%

244) *The commonest cations and anions found in the ECF are:*

   a) $K^+ + Cl$
   b) $Na^+ + Cl$
   c) $Ca^2 + HCO_2$
   d) $Mg^{2+} + Cl$

245) *Which ONE of the following is the largest fluid compartment in the body?*

   a) Extracellular fluid
   b) Interstitial fluid
   c) Intracellular fluid
   d) Plasma water

246) *Inevitable or insensible fluid loss occurs through which ONE of these routes?*

   a) The gastrointestinal tract
   b) The respiratory tract
   c) The urinary tract
   d) In vomitus

247) *What percentage of the total body water is contained within the intracellular fluid?*

   a) 25%
   b) 40%
   c) 60%
   d) 75%

248) *A 5% solution contains which ONE of the following?*

   a) 5 g of solute in 100 ml of solvent
   b) 5 g of solvent in 100 ml of solute
   c) 5 g of solute in 1000 ml of solvent
   d) 5 g of solvent in 1000 ml of solute

249) *Which ONE of the following cations is present in greatest abundance in the intracellular fluid?*

a) Calcium
b) Magnesium
c) Potassium
d) Sodium

250) *Which two ions are present in greatest abundance in plasma?*

a) Potassium and chloride
b) Potassium and phosphate
c) Sodium and bicarbonate
d) Sodium and chloride

251) *What is the volume of water required per 24 hours to maintain normal water balance in a healthy dog?*

a) 10–20 ml/kg
b) 40–60 ml/kg
c) 80–120 ml/kg
d) 150–200 ml/kg

252) *What is the normal volume of urine produced by a healthy dog in 24 hours?*

a) 10 ml/kg
b) 20 ml/kg
c) 50 ml/kg
d) 100 ml/kg

253) *What is the normal range of blood pH in the dog?*

    a) 7.00–7.20

    b) 7.00–7.50

    c) 7.15–7.25

    d) 7.35–7.45

254) *Which ONE of the following is a crystalloid solution?*

    a) Dextran 70

    b) Haemaccel

    c) 0.9% sodium chloride

    d) Whole blood

255) *Into which anticoagulant is blood for transfusion normally collected?*

    a) Acid citrate dextrose

    b) EDTA

    c) Fluoride

    d) Heparin

256) *Which ONE of the following combinations of ions below are the principal ions in Hartmann's solution?*

    a) Sodium, chloride, bicarbonate

    b) Sodium, chloride, bicarbonate, potassium

    c) Sodium, potassium

    d) Potassium, phosphate, bicarbonate

257) *What is the normal range of central venous pressure in a healthy dog?*

a) 3–7 cm H_2O
b) 3–7 mmHg
c) 10–15 cm H_2O
d) 10–15 mmHg

258) *At what percentage dehydration does loss of skin elasticity occur in the dehydrated animal?*

a) 2%
b) 5%
c) 7%
d) 12%

259) *Which ONE of the following fluids is hypertonic with respect to body fluid?*

a) Dextran 70
b) Haemaccel
c) 0.18% sodium chloride with 4% dextrose
d) 0.9% sodium chloride

260) *Which ONE of the following conditions is most likely to lead to metabolic alkalosis?*

a) Apnoea
b) Diarrhoea
c) Vomiting
d) Diabetic crisis

261) *A 10-kg dog is put onto intravenous fluids at a rate of 1.5 times maintenance (maintenance = 50 ml/kg/ 24 h). What is the total daily volume it needs and how many drips per minute should you set if the giving set delivers 20 drops/ml?*

    a) 500: 7 drops per minute
    b) 750: 10 drops per minute
    c) 500: 10 drops per minute
    d) 750: 7 drops per minute

262) *A burette giving set is often used to administer fluids to small dogs and cats because:*

    a) fluids can be given faster than using a conventional giving set
    b) small volumes can be given accurately
    c) the apparatus heats the fluid
    d) the vein is more likely to stay patent

263) *Central venous pressure measures the pressure in the:*

    a) left atrium
    b) left ventricle
    c) right atrium
    d) right ventricle

264) *A 12.5-kg mongrel has been vomiting for 3 days and is estimated to be 8% dehydrated. What approximate fluid volume should you give to rehydrate this dog?*

   a) 500 ml
   b) 1000 ml
   c) 2000 ml
   d) 2240 ml

265) *Which ONE of the following solutions would you give intravenously to maintain an animal once it had been rehydrated?*

   a) Hartmann's solution
   b) Plasma
   c) 5% dextrose
   d) 0.18% sodium chloride, 4% dextrose

266) *If you wished to maintain a 36-kg dog on a drip and you needed to give 2160 ml over 24 hours, how fast would you set the drip? (Assume that 1 ml = 20 drops.)*

   a) 1 drop per second
   b) 1 drop every 2 seconds
   c) 1 drop every 3 seconds
   d) 2 drops per second

267) *The type of body water which makes up about 5% of the animal's total body weight is:*

a) intracellular fluid
b) extracellular fluid
c) plasma
d) synovial fluid

268) *Which ONE of the following conditions would result in a primary water deficit?*

a) Unconsciousness
b) Vomiting
c) Diarrhoea
d) Burns

269) *The anticoagulant which is used when collecting blood for blood transfusion is:*

a) acid citrate dextrose (ACD)
b) heparin
c) EDTA
d) fluoride oxalate

270) *Central venous pressure provides an indication of the state of an animal's circulation. What is the normal central venous pressure in small animals?*

a) 3–7 cm water
b) 150–160 mm water
c) 3–7 mmHg
d) 150–160 mmHg

271) *Which ONE of the following is hypertonic with respect to plasma?*

   a) Dextran 70
   b) Haemaccel
   c) 0.18%NaCl with 4% dextrose
   d) 0.9% NaCl

272) *How is inevitable fluid lost?*

   a) In vomitus
   b) The gastro-intestinal tract
   c) The respiratory tract
   d) The urinary tract

273) *How much of an adult dog's total body weight is water?*

   a) 40%
   b) 60%
   c) 20%
   d) 15%

274) *Which ONE of the following is found within the cells of body tissues?*

   a) Transcellular fluid
   b) Plasma water
   c) Interstitial fluid
   d) Intracellular fluids

275) *Which ONE of the following is found in the spaces between the cells?*

a) Transcellular fluid
b) Plasma water
c) Interstitial fluid
d) Intracellular fluids

276) *Which ONE of the following is found within the vascular compartments?*

a) Transcellular fluid
b) Plasma water
c) Interstitial fluid
d) Intracellular fluids

277) *Plasma contains which ONE of the following as its main cation?*

a) Potassium
b) Sodium
c) Chloride
d) Magnesium

278) *Plasma contains which ONE of the following as its main anion?*

a) Potassium
b) Sodium
c) Chloride
d) Magnesium

279) *Which ONE of the following is classed as an 'inevitable' water loss?*

   a) Water lost through excretion of faeces
   b) Water lost through excretion of urine
   c) Water lost through excretion of vomiting
   d) Water lost via the respiratory tract

280) *An animal can suffer 'primary water depletion' through having the condition diabetes insipidus. Which ONE of the following is also a source of primary water depletion?*

   a) Prolonged inappetance
   b) Vomiting
   c) Diarrhoea
   d) Wound drainage

281) *Potassium depletion can occur from which ONE of the following conditions?*

   a) Acute renal failure
   b) Urethral obstruction
   c) Addison's disease
   d) Vomiting

282) *If an animal is urinating at a rate of 0.4 ml/kg/h you could say it was suffering from:*

   a) oliguria
   b) dysuria
   c) polyuria
   d) anuria

283) *Respiratory alkalosis can be caused by:*

   a) impaired ventilation
   b) over ventilation
   c) increased levels of carbon dioxide
   d) cerebral oedema

284) *The volume of blood which can be collected from a dog for a transfusion is:*

   a) 5–10 ml/kg
   b) 10–20 ml/kg
   c) 15–25ml/kg
   d) 20–30ml/kg

285) *The volume of blood which can be collected from a cat for a transfusion is:*

   a) 20 ml
   b) 30 ml
   c) 40 ml
   d) 50 ml

286) *In which ONE of the following anticoagulants would you store blood at 4% for 4 weeks?*

   a) Acid citrate dextrose
   b) Citrate phosphate dextrose
   c) Ethylene diamine tetra acid
   d) Lithium heparin

287) *Which ONE of the following is NOT a type of vasculogenic shock?*

   a) Neurogenic shock
   b) Hypovolaemic shock
   c) Endotoxic shock
   d) Anaphylactic shock

288) *How much fluid should you give a 25-kg dog over 24 hours for maintenance?*

   a) 1000 ml
   b) 1250 ml
   c) 1500 ml
   d) 1750 ml

289) *A 6-kg cat has a PCV of 45%. What is the fluid deficit (assuming the baseline is 50%)?*

   a) 1200 ml
   b) 900 ml
   c) 600 ml
   d) 300 ml

290) *A 20-kg dog has a known PCV of 38%. It is now dehydrated and its PCV is 56%. What is the fluid deficit?*

   a) 2700
   b) 3000
   c) 3300
   d) 3600

291) *How many drops/ml does a normal giving set usually deliver?*

   a) 15–20 drops/ml
   b) 20–30 drops/ml
   c) 50 drops/ml
   d) 60 drops/ml

292) *A 12-kg dog has a known PCV of 45%. Its PCV is now 55%. How many ml of fluid per minute would you give the patient over a 24-hour period?*

   a) 0.80 ml per minute
   b) 1.25 ml per minute
   c) 1.65 ml per minute
   d) 2.10 ml per minute

293) *Using a giving set that delivers 20 drops per ml, what will the flow rate be for a 25-kg dog over 24 hours, assuming a maintenance requirement of 50 ml/kg/24 hours?*

   a) Approximately 1 drop per 12 seconds
   b) Approximately 1 drop per 5 seconds
   c) Approximately 1 drop per 3 seconds
   d) Approximately 1 drop per 1 second

294) *Plasma can be stored for 6 months at:*

   a) −70°C
   b) −50°C
   c) −40°C
   d) −30°C

295) *Which ONE of the following fluids is hypertonic in respect to plasma?*

   a) Ringer's solution
   b) Haemaccel
   c) 5% dextrose
   d) Dextrans

296) *Which ONE of the following fluids would be best to rehydrate a patient who is suffering from post-gastric losses?*

   a) 0.9% sodium chloride
   b) Ringer's lactate
   c) 0.18% sodium chloride in 4% dextrose
   d) sodium bicarbonate

297) *A dehydrated 20-kg dog is placed on an intravenous drip at 1.5 times maintenance (assume maintenance is 50 ml/kg/day). What is the total daily volume required and what should the drip rate be if the giving set delivers 20 drops/ml?*

   a) 1500 ml total, at approx 21 drops per minute
   b) 1500 ml total, at approx 10 drops per minute
   c) 750 ml total, at approx 21 drops per minute
   d) 750 ml total, at approx 10 drops per minute

298) *A dehydrated dog weighing 10 kg is placed on a drip at 2 times maintenance for 24 hours (assume maintenance is 50 ml/kg/day). Assume the giving set delivers 20 drops/ml, how often should a drop be delivered?*

a) Every 13–14 seconds
b) Every 7–8 seconds
c) Every 5–6 seconds
d) Every 3–4 seconds

299) *A dehydrated 4-kg cat is placed on intravenous fluids at 1.5 times maintenance for 24 hours (assume maintenance is 50 ml/kg/day). What is the total volume of fluid requested, and what would the drip rate be if the giving set delivers 15 drops/ml?*

a) 150 ml total, at approx 3 drops per minute
b) 300 ml total, at approx 6 drops per minute
c) 150 ml total, at approx 6 drops per minute
d) 300 ml total, at approx 3 drops per minute

300) *An RTA animal weighing 10 kg is to be treated with 1-hour fluids for 24 hours at maintenance rate. What is the drop rate selected if the giving set administers 20 drops per ml?*

a) Approx 2–3 drop/min
b) Approx 4–5 drops/min
c) Approx 6–7 drops/min
d) Approx 7–8 drops/min

Answers

1)	b	23)	a	45)	d	67)	c
2)	c	24)	d	46)	c	68)	b
3)	c	25)	b	47)	b	69)	a
4)	a	26)	a	48)	c	70)	c
5)	d	27)	d	49)	a	71)	b
6)	c	28)	b	50)	d	72)	b
7)	a	29)	a	51)	b	73)	d
8)	d	30)	c	52)	b	74)	d
9)	b	31)	b	53)	d	75)	b
10)	c	32)	c	54)	b	76)	c
11)	d	33)	b	55)	c	77)	a
12)	a	34)	b	56)	a	78)	c
13)	b	35)	d	57)	b	79)	d
14)	c	36)	a	58)	a	80)	c
15)	b	37)	d	59)	c	81)	a
16)	c	38)	c	60)	d	82)	b
17)	d	39)	a	61)	a	83)	c
18)	d	40)	d	62)	b	84)	c
19)	c	41)	a	63)	c	85)	a
20)	c	42)	a	64)	b	86)	c
21)	a	43)	c	65)	b	87)	d
22)	b	44)	b	66)	a	88)	d

89)	b	125)	a	161)	a	197)	b
90)	a	126)	d	162)	c	198)	c
91)	c	127)	b	163)	b	199)	d
92)	b	128)	d	164)	b	200)	c
93)	d	129)	b	165)	a	201)	d
94)	d	130)	a	166)	b	202)	b
95)	d	131)	b	167)	c	203)	d
96)	a	132)	c	168)	b	204)	a
97)	b	133)	d	169)	d	205)	b
98)	d	134)	a	170)	b	206)	a
99)	d	135)	a	171)	a	207)	d
100)	a	136)	a	172)	d	208)	c
101)	a	137)	d	173)	b	209)	d
102)	c	138)	a	174)	b	210)	d
103)	b	139)	b	175)	b	211)	b
104)	c	140)	d	176)	a	212)	c
105)	c	141)	b	177)	c	213)	a
106)	a	142)	b	178)	a	214)	c
107)	d	143)	a	179)	a	215)	b
108)	b	144)	d	180)	c	216)	b
109)	a	145)	c	181)	d	217)	d
110)	a	146)	d	182)	a	218)	a
111)	a	147)	c	183)	b	219)	a
112)	c	148)	a	184)	b	220)	d
113)	b	149)	c	185)	d	221)	c
114)	b	150)	d	186)	b	222)	b
115)	b	151)	b	187)	a	223)	c
116)	d	152)	b	188)	b	224)	a
117)	b	153)	a	189)	d	225)	a
118)	b	154)	c	190)	c	226)	d
119)	d	155)	d	191)	d	227)	a
120)	a	156)	b	192)	d	228)	c
121)	b	157)	c	193)	a	229)	c
122)	a	158)	a	194)	a	230)	a
123)	a	159)	b	195)	a	231)	b
124)	c	160)	a	196)	b	232)	a

233)	d	250)	d	267)	c	284)	b
234)	d	251)	b	268)	a	285)	c
235)	a	252)	b	269)	a	286)	b
236)	c	253)	d	270)	a	287)	c
237)	c	254)	c	271)	a	288)	b
238)	d	255)	a	272)	c	289)	c
239)	a	256)	b	273)	b	290)	d
240)	b	257)	a	274)	d	291)	a
241)	d	258)	b	275)	c	292)	a
242)	a	259)	a	276)	b	293)	c
243)	d	260)	c	277)	b	294)	a
244)	b	261)	b	278)	c	295)	d
245)	c	262)	b	279)	d	296)	b
246)	b	263)	c	280)	a	297)	a
247)	b	264)	b	281)	d	298)	d
248)	a	265)	d	282)	a	299)	d
249)	c	266)	b	283)	b	300)	c